Ícaro Fernando Fonsêca Braga
Beatriz Stransky
Danylo de Araujoo Viana

Modelling the effects of genetic alterations

Ícaro Fernando Fonsêca Braga
Beatriz Stransky
Danylo de Araujoo Viana

Modelling the effects of genetic alterations

In tumour progression

ScienciaScripts

Imprint

Cover image: www.ingimage.com

This book is a translation from the original published under ISBN 978-613-9-66981-3.

Publisher:
Sciencia Scripts
is a trademark of
Dodo Books Indian Ocean Ltd. and OmniScriptum S.R.L publishing group

120 High Road, East Finchley, London, N2 9ED, United Kingdom
Str. Armeneasca 28/1, office 1, Chisinau MD-2012, Republic of Moldova, Europe
Printed at: see last page
ISBN: 978-620-8-11543-2

To my family, who over the years have never stopped believing in my potential. Especially my mum, Sônia Fonsêca, who has never stopped trying to support me in my decisions and who has always taught me to think of others before myself. Without you, none of this would have been possible.

ACKNOWLEDGEMENTS

To God for the gift of life, without his presence I would be nothing.

To my family, who have always believed in me in every struggle I have fought. My mum, Sônia, for all her love, of which I will never be worthy enough. My grandmother, Isaura, my uncle and cousin, Sóstenes and Firmo, my aunt and cousins, Solange, Karla, Kalyanne and Kyara. A family that, even in the midst of problems, still finds room to smile.

To my girlfriend, Moema, who even when I was sad never gave up on me or motivated me.

To the DeMolay Order, which has taught me since I was fourteen how to be a better and worthy person. Without the lessons I learnt there, I would be half the man I am today. At this point, I would like to quote one of our most beautiful ceremonies, that of the Lights.

However, each of you carries within your heart a flame, a torch to guide you through the darkness. If you can make this light shine on someone else, if you can penetrate the depths of their soul and ignite the flame that is there, then that is your purpose in living."

To the entire Clinical Engineering team at Onofre Lopes University Hospital, who never thought twice before teaching me something. In particular, Rafael, who believed in my potential and gave me the opportunity to participate effectively in the team.

To my friends and partners at Airmid, who have shared many burdens with me throughout this year. This company has a long future.

To all my friends, I just have to thank God for putting me in your path.

To my supervisors, Beatriz Stransky and Marcus Nunes, who at no time spared any effort to help me complete this work. Beatriz, who believed in me since January and entrusted me with this line of research, and Marcus, who, since becoming my co-supervisor, has never stopped adding to my work. This is our achievement and there is still much to come.

Along with the supervisors is the entire BioMe team, Professor Sandro Souza, Vandeclecio, Jorge and André, who each contributed their own area of expertise to the development and completion of this final year's work.

Finally, to all the teachers who have been with me since I was a child and who have moulded me into the citizen I am today.

SUMMARY

SUMMARY

Genetic alterations that predispose an individual to a particular cancer have been identified in studies carried out on a genome-wide scale. Cancer is the result of genetic alterations that give it adaptive advantages, such as the ability to metastasise. In this context, the successive mutations resulting from tumour growth provide an increase in the adaptive advantage of the cell that undergoes these mutations and result in the expansion of cancer. However, our understanding of aspects relating to the dynamics of replication, survival and evolution of the tumour cell population has not yet reached the level of the advances made in molecular genetics. In this final project, we used a mathematical model based on the stochastic *branching* process capable of relating tumour growth to the addition of *driver* mutations, *which are* responsible for this tumour growth, and to *passenger* mutations, which have no influence on growth. Using this model, we compared the simulation results with genomic data from samples in the DB Mutation database of the Interdisciplinary Bioinformatics Centre at the Federal University of Rio Grande do Norte. After running 100,000 simulations on the Instituto Metrópole Digital cluster, we obtained results that are similar to the current literature on evolutionary dynamics. Our results support the premise that after acquiring around four *driver* mutations, the tumour will be skilful enough to adapt to the organism, making it difficult to die. We also observed that the number of *passengers* resulting from successive *driver* mutations increases as the *driver* mutations increase, but that after a certain time they stabilise at 29 *passengers,* due to the proposed simulation time. We hope that the introduction of genomic data into the mathematical model will generate new information and hypotheses about the evolutionary dynamics of tumours and make it possible to model experimental treatment applications in a simulated environment in the future.

Keywords: Cancer. Evolutionary dynamics. Stochastic modelling. *Drirerr.* **mutation**.

CHAPTER 1

INTRODUCTION

According to the *World Cancer Report 2014* of the *International Agency for Research on Cancer, an* arm of the World Health Organisation, the premise that cancer is a public health problem is unquestionable. In the coming decades, cancer in the population is expected to account for 80 per cent of the more than 20 million new cases estimated for 2025 (INCA, 2014).

After hundreds of years of advances in science, it is possible to observe the amount of information acquired in cancer research, revealing it as a disease based on changes in the genome. Although there is no concrete inaugural scientific record of the disease, there are mentions of Egyptians, Persians and Indians who identified malignant tumours (STRATTON, 2009). The basis of all research lies in the discovery of alterations in genes that modify the function of the gene product - the protein, and which generate a gain or loss of function in the protein. This gain or loss of function is related to the acquisition of milestones that the tumour needs in order to proliferate. These behaviours have been identified through observations of alterations in human and animal cancer cells (STRATTON, 2009).

Cancer can originate from alterations caused by internal factors, such as a genetic mutation inherited from one of the parents, and external factors, caused by some mutagenic environmental agent, both of which can lead to an increase in cell replication. At the beginning of tumour development, the cell initially does not have a high adaptive advantage, and the transformation process is slow and dependent on the emergence of new mutations that will, over time, guarantee the survival of the tumour. However, after accumulating a sufficient number of mutations, this cell will have an advantage over the others. As well as proliferating

faster, these modifications may confer other abilities that provide it with better adaptation and growth, such as evading signs of cell apoptosis or vascularisation of the tumour (HANAHAN; WEINBERG, 2000).

Thus, a key point of research today is to distinguish between the emergence of *driver-type* **mutations, which confer an adaptive advantage on the cell, and** *passenger* **mutations (neutral mutations), which do not have this effect (BOZIC; NOWAK, 2010). However, current methods have yielded poor results when trying to model the dynamics of a tumour population in view of genetic alterations, such as**

for example, the Wright-Fisher approach, which uses a random perspective that does not evaluate the additional replication gain of cells with each new *driver* **mutation (BEERENWINKEL et al, 2007).**

Investigating this successive gain of adaptive advantage and its effect on cancer progression is what motivates this research. A cell with a *driver* **mutation at the start of a tumourigenic process has little adaptive value, but it does produce alterations in tumour growth that could lead to a new mutation more easily. Therefore, with each new** *driver* **mutation, there will be a gain in replication and, consequently, an increase in the possibility of new mutations. This will confer a new adaptive factor, such as inefficient signalling for cell apoptosis. It is clear that with each new** *driver* **mutation, there will be a new change in the adaptive quality of the tumour, corroborating its expansion (STRATTON** *et al,* **2009).**

This work consists of implementing a model capable of simulating the evolutionary dynamics of cancer based on its **driver** mutations and comparing the simulation data with real data obtained from sequencing and analysing **patients**' genomes. The study was based on research carried out by Bozic in 2010, where using a stochastic model it was possible to better understand the role of **driver** mutations in the adaptive advantage and growth of tumours. To compare our simulation data, we also carried out a study with real data from the DB Mutation database.

CHAPTER 2

OBJECTIVES

2.1 GENERAL

To implement a mathematical-computational model of evolutionary dynamics, capable of simulating tumour growth progression, in order to evaluate the influence of *driver-type* mutations on tumour growth.

2.2 SPECIFIC

The specific objectives are:

- **Implement the mathematical model in a computer environment;**
- **Simulate the dynamics of tumour growth using parameters related to breast cancer - such as u, mutation acquisition rate; v, neutral mutation acquisition rate, *s,* adaptive advantage, T, folding time (iteration) and *t,* number of iterations between t_0 and the start of the last lineage;**
- **Analysing breast tumour genomes from the DB Mutation database;**
- **Compare the simulation results with information obtained from bioinformatic analysis (DB Mutation data) in relation to the proportion of *passenger* and *drive* mutations.**

CHAPTER 3

LITERATURE REVIEW

This section presents a bibliographical review of the most relevant topics in this work. The subjects covered here will contribute to a better understanding of the content that will be presented in the following topics. The first part of this section will present a review of cancer, highlighting the effects of genetic changes on the tumour growth process. This will be followed by a discussion of the statistical method on which this modelling was based, including aspects of its theory and modelling.

3.1 Cancer

Cancer has received a lot of attention over the years due to its high incidence in the population. The global estimate carried out in 2012 by the Globocan/Iarc project showed that of the estimated 14 million new cases, more than 60 per cent occurred in developing countries. For mortality, the situation is even worse, as it was found that of the 8 million deaths predicted, 70 per cent occurred in these same countries (IARC, 2014). The most common types of cancer in the world were lung (1.8 million), breast (1.7 million), bowel (1.4 million) and prostate (1.1 million). In men, the most frequent cancers were lung, prostate, bowel, stomach and liver. In women, breast, bowel, cervical, lung and stomach cancers were among the most common.

Estimates in Brazil (Figure 1 and Table 1) for the 2016/2017 biennium point to around 600,000 new cases of cancer. This profile is similar to that of Latin America and the Caribbean, where most countries are also developing. As a result, we are seeing a public health problem, where this disease is becoming increasingly common as the population's life expectancy increases (INCA, 2016).

Table 2 - Estimated number of cancer cases in 2016 in Brazil (INCA, 2016).

Primary localisation Malignant neoplasm	Estimated New Cases			1				
	Men		StatesCapitals		Women Capital		States	
	Cases	Gross rate	Cases	Gross rate	Cases	Gross rate	Cases	Gross Rate
Prostate	61.200	61.82	13.940	64.93	-	-	-	
Mama Femirwia	-	-	-	-	57.960	56,20	18.990	79,37
Cervix	-	-	-	-	16.340	15,85	4.550	19,07
Trachea. Bronchus and Lungs	17.330	17.49	4.430	20,59	10.89 0	10,54	3.230	13,49
Colon and rectum	16.66 0	16.84	5.560	25,80	17.62 0	17,10	6.210	25,95
Stomach	12.020	13.04	3.130	14,54	7.600	7,37	2.180	9.07
Oral Cavity	11.140	11,27	2.780	12,95	4.350	4.21	1.230	5,04
Larynx	6.360	6,43	1.600	7,50	990	0,94	320	0,97
Bladder	7.200	7.26	2.110	9,79	2.470	2,39	830	3,21
Oesophagus	7.950	8.04	1.460	6.75	2.860	2,76	610	2,27
Ovado	-		-		6.150	5,95	2.170	8,92
Hodgkin's lymphoma	1.460	1,46	450	1.74	1.010	0,93	400	1,33
Non-Hodgkin's lymphoma	5.210	5.27	1.550	7.15	5.030	4,88	1.670	7,02
GlándiJa Thyroid	1.090	1,00	350	1.27	5.870	5.70	1.800	7,46
Central Nervous System	5.440	5,50	1.290	5,86	4.830	4.68	1.250	5,20
Leukaemias	5.540	5,63	1.370	6,38	4.530	4,38	1.180	4.88
Jtero's body	-		-		6.950	6,74	2.530	10,47
Skin Melanoma	3.000	3,03	840	3,86	2.670	2,59	740	2.96
Other locations	51.050	52.38	11.890	55,45	47.840	46.36	11.82 0	49.33
Subtotal	214.350	216.48	52.750	245,63	205.960	199,57	61.710	257,55
Fish not Melanoma	60.850	81.66	17.370	80,90	94.910	91,98	21.910	91,65
All Keoplasms	295.200	298.13	70.120	326,51	300.870	291,54	83.62 0	348, 99|

* Numbers rounded up to multiples of 10.

Table 2 - Distribution of the ten most common types of cancer estimated for 2016 by sex

(INCA, 2016).

Primary Localisation	Cases	%	Men	Women	Primary Localisation	Cases	%
Pnistafa	61.200	26.6%			Female breast	57.960	26.1%
Trachea. Bronchus and Lung	17.330	6,1%			Cúkin eReto	17.620	6,6%
Colon and rectum	16.660	7.6%			Cervix	16.340	7,9%
Stomach	12.920	6.0%			Trachea. Bronchus and Lung	10.690	5.3%
Oral Cavity	11.140	5.2%			Stomach	7.600	3.7%
Oesophagus	7.950	3.7%			Body of the uterus	6.950	3,4%
Bengo	7.200	3.4%			Ovárki	6.150	3,0%
Larynx	6.360	3,0%			Thyroid Gland	5.870	2,9%
Leukaemias	5.540	2.6%			Non-Hodgkin's lymphoma	5.030	2,4%
Central Nervous System	5.440	2.5%			Central Nervous System	4.830	2,3%

'Numbers rounded to multiples of 10

3.2Cancer as an evolutionary process

Some lines of research show that tumour development is a process made up of several stages and that these stages reflect genetic changes that lead to the progressive transformation of normal cells into tumours. These transformations are caused by mutations that occur stochastically. These mutations can be classified according to their influence on the establishment and development of the tumour. **Driver-type** mutations guarantee cells greater adaptability and survival in the organism, and with each new **driver** mutation we can

observe an increase in the tumour's adaptive advantage. **Passenger-type** mutations have no effect (RENAN, 1993).

In addition, we can observe a behaviour where with each new **driver** mutation, the time required for a new mutation to occur is shorter (Figure 1). Therefore, the interdependence of the number of **driver** mutations and tumour growth is a fact.

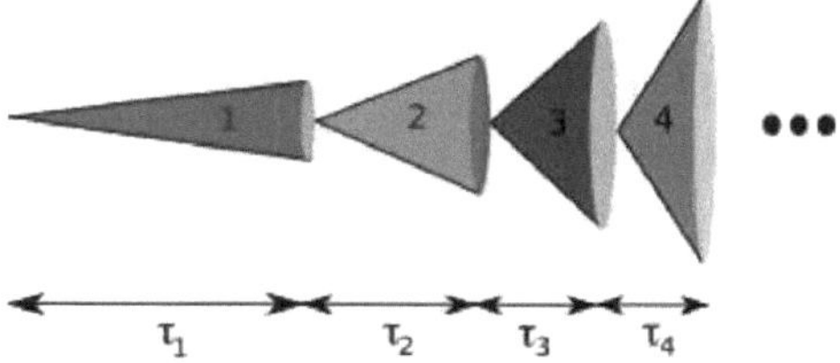

Figura 1 - **Time needed for a new driver mutation (BOZIC et al., 2010).**

In this context, researchers have listed a number of capabilities that a mutated cell can acquire for its adaptation (HAHN et al., 1999). These are sustained by the new mutations that occur from the first mutation and which give the tumour a high adaptive advantage (Figure 2).

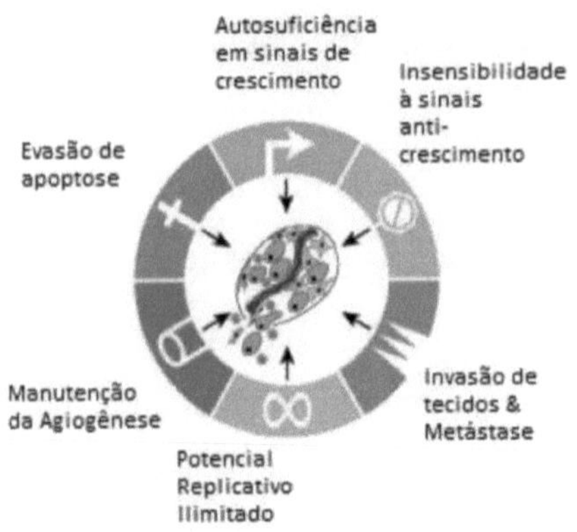

Figura 2 - **Acquired capacities of cancer (adapted from HANAHAN et al., 2000).**

1.1.1 Self-sufficiency in growth signals

Normal cells require growth signals before they can change from a state of quiescence - a state in which the cell is metabolically active but not proliferating - to an active state of proliferation. These signals are transmitted to the cell by transmembrane receptors that bind different classes of signalling: growth factors, extracellular matrix components and cell-cell adhesion/interaction molecules. There is no normal cell type in nature that can proliferate without the presence of growth factors. Many oncogenes, genes related to the appearance of tumours, act by mimicking exacerbated growth signalling behaviour (HANAHAN; WEINBERG, 2000).

1.1.2 Insensitivity to anti-growth signals

In normal tissue, multiple anti-proliferative signals operate to maintain cell quiescence and homeostasis. However, cancer cells are able to evade these signals in order to continue their growth. The cells act by directly altering their replication cycle, going unnoticed by these signals

(HANAHAN; WEINBERG, 2000).

1.1.3 Evasion of apoptosis

The ability of tumour cells to expand is linked not only to their ability to proliferate, but also to their ability to prevent programmed cell death - apoptosis. Apoptosis occurs when the environment or internal factors send signals for cells to die, as they are unable to carry out their functions properly. Therefore, an expanding tumour must overcome this barrier in order to render these programmed death signals non-functional (HANAHAN; WEINBERG, 2000).

1.1.4 Unlimited replication potential

The capacities explained above could alone constitute the necessary advantages for the complete growth of a tumour, however recent studies have shown that this disordered growth and evasion of the communication between cells that generates apoptosis, in itself, is not enough to guarantee tumour growth. One example is breast cancer, where many and perhaps all types of breast cells carry an autonomous programme that limits their growth. This programme operates independently of intercellular connections, thus constituting yet another barrier to be overcome so that the tumour becomes macroscopic and lethal (HANAHAN; WEINBERG, 2000).

1.1.5 Maintenance of angiogenesis

A major barrier to tumour growth lies in the fact that at a certain point in its growth it becomes very large. The bloodstream, and consequently nutrients, cannot reach the inside of the tumour and cells can enter a process of necrosis. In order to stay alive, the tumour must create blood channels that reach its interior and bring food and oxygen to the cells. Once this barrier is broken, the tumour will work as a self-sufficient organism (HANAHAN; WEINBERG, 2013).

1.1.6 Tissue invasion & Metastasis

Finally, after successive increases in its adaptive advantage, the tumour can invade other tissues and spread throughout the body. This process is known as metastasis, where the cancer cells, now with a high adaptive value, can detach from the original tissue, migrate via the blood or lymphatic circulation and establish new tumour foci in other parts of the body (HANAHAN; WEINBERG, 2013).

3.3 Cancer Genome

Like all the cells in our body, cancer cells are direct descendants of mitotic divisions and therefore carry a copy of their genetic code. However, this DNA that cancer cells carry has a number of differences from its progenitor, due to mutations and other alterations in the cell's genome.

These alterations include base substitutions, insertions or deletions of small or large segments of DNA, rearrangements of broken segments in other parts of the genome, etc. These alterations can be the result of various factors such as genetic predisposition from the parents or caused by external factors, such as sunburn that induces skin cancer.

One point to bear in mind is that all cancers are the result of mutations, but not every mutation is involved in the development of cancer. To this end, it is necessary to introduce the concept of **driver-type** mutations and **passenger-type** mutations.

A **driver** mutation is closely related to the process of oncogenesis, it gives cancer an increase in its adaptive advantage and increases its growth. **Passenger** mutations, on the other hand, do not give the cancer an increase in growth and therefore have no influence on its development. They are mutations that result from the process of tumourigenesis and their number usually increases in line with the increase in **driver** mutations.

3.4 Models of Cancer Evolutionary Dynamics

Evolutionary dynamics models help to understand how tumours develop and can play an essential role in establishing prognosis and predicting the results of medical interventions (WACLAW et al, 2015). An example of this is in target-focused therapy, in which medication is released at the target site (tumour), where it can be most effective. Bozic et al. developed a density-dependent tumour growth model, and taking tumour size into account, it was possible to identify that both tumour growth and the distribution of daughter cells are limited by geometry and metabolic factors. In this sense, mathematical models have been an essential tool to inform which combination of therapies can minimise cancer resistance (BOZIC et al, 2013).

In 2013, Bozic and colleagues presented a mathematical model capable of describing the evolutionary dynamics of lesions in response to treatment. Twenty melanoma patients were studied and the characteristics were reproduced and they underwent treatment in different modalities (sequential, simultaneous, different drug combinations, etc.). It was identified that often the best combined and simultaneous treatment with two drugs is quite effective in controlling the disease, and that in cases of greater need, more aggressive tumours, a good option would be the application of up to three drugs.

In the same vein, various mathematical models have been developed and computationally implemented to help understand and test hypotheses about the biology of cancer. The Multistage Theory is based on the probability of cancer developing with age, but this method does not look at the kinetics of tumour creation and progression, considering only that there are stages that must be reached during tumour growth (ARMITAGE, 1954).

Subsequently, it was observed that the most interesting methodology for modelling evolutionary dynamics was stochastic models, where the behaviour is very close to the biological behaviour of mutations, i.e. random, with no deterministic characteristics without a biological basis. Stochastic models have been developed for both mixed populations and structured populations, where it is possible to implement different parameters (NOWAK, 2006).

There are still deterministic models, where it is possible, through dynamic systems, to describe the average behaviour of evolutionary systems, which are easier to implement, but can neglect the random character that exists in biology (BEERENWINKEL et al, 2014).

Among the studies carried out, a more appropriate proposition is that tumour evolution is closely linked to the number of **driver** mutations the tumour has, as they give the tumour the adaptive advantage capable of overcoming the barriers described above. In this way, their number represents a major adaptive advantage for cancer. Thus, an interesting example of a mathematical model based on the stochastic nature of biology and which also translates a relationship between **driver** mutations and **passenger** mutations is the model proposed by Bozic in 2010. In this model, cancer biology parameters were established and simulations were carried out according to these parameters. At the end, the simulated data was compared with the real data, pancreatic cancer and gliobastoma, in relation to the proportion of cells with **driver** and *passenger* mutations, *and* the CHASM **(Cancer-specific High-throughput Annotation of Somatic Mutations)** filter (CARTER, 2009) was used to classify the *drivers*. It was found that both graphs have a similar behaviour with a logarithmic curve, and that as a result of the increase in *driver* mutations there was also an increase in *passenger* mutations (BOZIC et al., 2010).

3.5 Galton-Watson stochastic model

The Galton-Watson process is a stochastic branching process that was first used to determine how long a family's surname would persist over generations. Due to its random characteristic, this method is of interest and adheres to research, since this method combines elements of a stochastic nature and it is possible to establish population growth parameters and separate them into possible outcomes.

Equation 2 - Basic equation of the Galton-Watson method.

$$X_{n+1} = \sum_{j=1}^{X_n} \xi_j^{(n)} \qquad \{\xi_j^{(n)} : n, j \in \mathbb{N}\}$$

In this equation we have X_n as the number of offspring (along the male line) of the nth generation and the number of male offspring of the jth line of these offspring.

In an attempt to estimate the lifespan of a family surname, the probability of each parent having no children (asexual), one child or two children was calculated. Therefore, using the branching methodology, the possible number of generations to which that surname could survive was estimated.

With this method it is possible to establish the probabilities related to certain behaviours (continuity, duplication, death) as exemplified in Figure 3. Later in the methodology of this work, we will identify the similarities of this situation with the probable scenarios of a cell division.

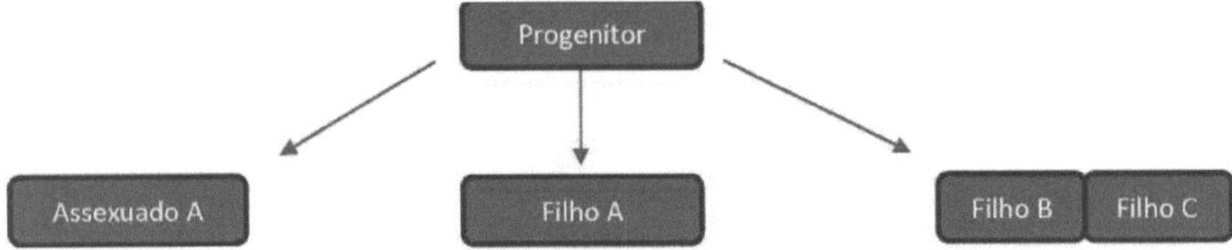

Figure 3 - Basic behaviour of a branching process.

CHAPTER 4

METHODOLOGY

The development of the project was organised into three macro-stages. These and their subdivisions are listed in the flowchart shown in Figure 4.

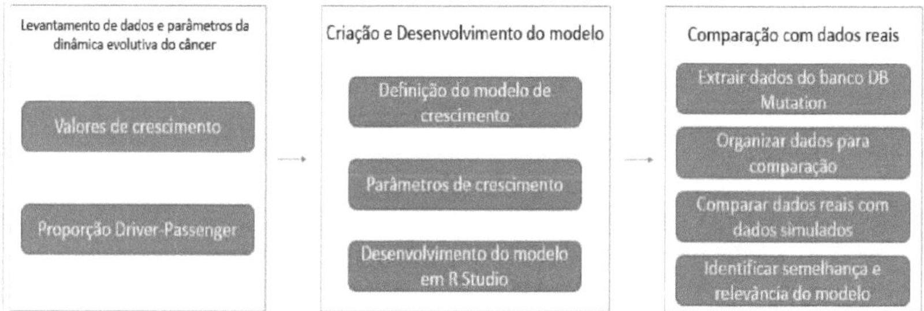

Figure 4 - Flowchart of the project stages.

4.1 Data collection and evolutionary dynamics parameters

In this study, it was necessary to acquire information on the evolutionary dynamics of cancer and its parameters. To this end, the literature was searched for representative values of tumour growth and the relationship between **driver** and **passenger** mutations.

4.1.1 Growth figures

For the model in question there are some parameters that influence the modelling, among them: point mutation rate, valid for any type of mutation, *driver* mutation rate - u, adaptive advantage - s, folding time (lifetime of a cell until the next division, our step) - T, number of *driver mutations - k,* number of *passenger mutations - n* and acquisition rate of neutral mutations - *v*.

Among these parameters, there are some considerations to be made. The point mutation rate has no applicability in our model. Since we want to observe the influence that *driver* mutations have on tumour growth, the use of this rate would imply the unnecessary observance of values such as *passenger* mutations.

As stated in the previous paragraph, the interest of this study lies in observing the consequences that **driver** mutations generate. As such, parameters such as the **driver** mutation rate, adaptive advantage and the number of **driver** mutations will be key factors in building the model. In addition, there are factors that must be taken into account, such as folding time and the rate of acquisition of neutral mutations, in order to count the **passenger** mutations that occurred during the simulation in the future.

4.1.2 Driver-Passenger ratio

Although the model is stochastic, the literature, according to our study, has not yet found a definitive model for determining the number of **passenger** mutations. This part of our model needs to be determined through an approximate calculation that will be made at the end of each simulation.

To do this, we'll use the following equation:

Equation 2 - Determining the number of *passenger* mutations.

$$n(t) = \frac{vt}{T}$$

In this equation, **n** is the total number of **passenger** mutations, **v** is the rate of acquisition of neutral mutations and **T** is the folding time. **T** and **v** are constant values and depend on the type of cancer being simulated, while **t** is dependent on the number of steps taken while the tumour exists.

4.2 Implementation and simulation

The model was generated in R Studio© software *(2016 The R Studio)* using parameters available in the literature and an auxiliary parallel computing package, since around 100,000 simulations were carried out with parameters for breast cancer. The simulations were run on a computer at the Metrópole Digital Institute in partnership with BioMe (Interdisciplinary Bioinformatics Centre) at the Federal University of Rio Grande do Norte. In addition, it was necessary to add limiting factors to the code such as total execution time and maximum understandable number of *driver* mutations.

4.2.1 Model - evolutionary dynamics

The dynamics of the evolutionary model of cancer, similar to the Galton-Watson model with the surnames, is based on three possible scenarios: generation of two daughter cells equal to the progenitor; generation of one daughter cell equal to the progenitor and another with a new **driver** mutation; and death. This can be seen in Figure 5 below:

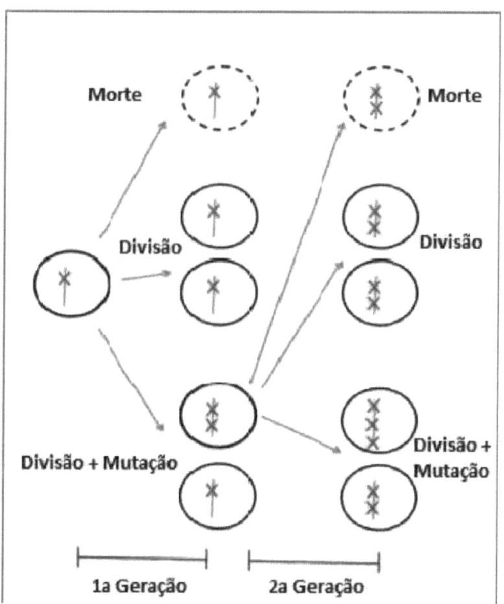

Figure 5 - Dynamics of tumour evolution and the possible results for each cell in

each iteration (adapted from ROGOES, 2010).

For the model in question, the probabilities of each event occurring are dependent on Equation 3, which represents the probability of a cell stagnating, there being no change in the total amount of the tumour, with **k** **driver** mutations, **s** being the initial adaptive advantage.

Equation 3 - Calculation of the probability of stagnation.

$$d_k = \frac{1}{2}(1 - s)^k$$

This probability, if s is equal to 0.04%, will be 49.8%. This means that the population of cells has a lower chance of dying or stagnating, thus maintaining its previous population size. It therefore has a 50.2 per cent chance of dividing into two new mutated cells.

4.2. 2Parameters

The parameter values were obtained from the literature and are listed in Table 3. The value for the acquisition rate of **driver** mutations was calculated by multiplying the acquisition rate of point mutations in tumours, $\sim 5 \times 10^{-10}$, by the number of positions in the genome that can become driver mutations, $\sim 3.4 \times 10^{4}$. In addition, a time limit was set for the simulation, and the time chosen was 20 years. This value has also been observed in the literature and represents a reliable interval for comparative analysis.

Due to the difficulty in determining the number of **passenger** mutations, it was decided that the code would count the steps taken until the last lineage was perpetuated. We will therefore use Equation 2 to estimate the number of **passenger** mutations from **t**, the number of steps for a given doubling time. Finally, we set the initial population to be just 1 cell with a

driver mutation.

Table 3 - Parameters and respective values used in the model.

Parameters	Breast cancer	Reference
Driver mutation rate	u = 3.4 x IO^{-5}	(BOZIC, 2010)
Adaptive advantage	s = 0,4% (0,004)	(BOZIC, 2010)
Bending time	T = 2 days	(DAI, 2015)
Acquisition rate of neutral mutations	v = 0,016	(BOZIC, 2010)
Initial population	1 cell	Chosen
Total simulation time	20 years	Chosen

4.3Bioinformatics

To assess the quality of the model, we compared the results obtained by the simulation with the results obtained by analysing the genomes available in the DB Mutation database.

4.3.1 DB Mutation database

The data for analysing the number of **driver** mutations and **passengers of** individuals was obtained from the DB MUTATION database, developed by BioMe (Interdisciplinary Bioinformatics Centre) at the Federal University of Rio Grande do Norte (BioInfo-IMD, 2016). DB Mutation includes information from the COSMIC (Catalogue of Somatic Mutations In Cancer) and TCGA (The Cancer Genome Atlas) databases. These databases contain sequencing samples from the most diverse types of cancer, and together they are the largest source of genome data currently available (THE SCIENTIST, 2012). Of these, we used 30 breast cancer samples from each bank.

DB Mutation adds some information by using a set of techniques to analyse whether the mutations found in each sample have an influence on tumour growth. The mutations are evaluated using nine parameters, called predictors, which are counted to form the NDamage indicator. If the mutation has passed at least five of them, the mutation is declared to be a **driver**. This study used these classification criteria to determine the **driver/passenger** ratios.

4.3.2Analysing genetic mutations using predictors

The parameters mentioned above are techniques that already exist in the literature. They come from dbNSFP, which is nothing more than a database that includes prediction mechanisms (LIU, 2013). These mechanisms generally look at characteristics such as sample sequence homogeneity, RNA and protein information, nucleotide substitution, etc. Many repeat each other's techniques, but it is believed that a ratio criterion of 5/9 effectively provides enough evidence to classify a mutation as a **driver** and if not, as a **passenger**. Table 4 briefly describes each of these predictors.

Table 4 - Predictors used in DB Mutation and their definitions (LIU, 2003).

Prediction mechanism	Evaluation factor
SIFT	It ranges from 0 to 1. Analyses the likelihood of a harmful effect from SNPs; the lower the score, the greater

	the likelihood of harm.
PolyPhen-2- HDIV	Automatic tool for predicting the possible impact of amino acid substitutions on the structure and function of human proteins. This prediction is based on the number of features included in the sequence, phylogenetic and structural information characterising the substitution.
PolyPhen-2- HVAR	Automatic tool for predicting the possible impact of amino acid substitutions on the structure and function of human proteins. This prediction is based on the number of features included in the sequence, phylogenetic and structural information characterising the substitution.
Mutation Taster	It employs a Bayes classifier to eventually predict the potential for a disease change. The Bayes classifier is fed with the results of all the tests and characteristics of the alterations and calculates the probabilities of alterations for an alteration being either a disease through mutation or a polymorphism with no effect.
Fathmm	Server capable of predicting the functional consequences of both coding variants and non-coding variants. Returns predictions capable of distinguishing between cancer promotion/driver mutations and other germline polymorphisms.
LTR	It is an efficient programme for finding complete LTR **retrotransposons** in gene sequences. It has a range of 0 to 1. It predicts

	whether a given mutation is deleterious (D), neutral (N) or undetermined (U), but these definitions are not based solely on the result value found.
MetaSVM	Support vector machine (SVM) determines a prediction result that incorporates ten other predictors (SIFT, PolyPhen-2 HDIV, Polyphen-2 HVAR, GERP++, MutationTaster, Mutation Assessor, FATHMM, LTR, SiPhy, PhyloP) and also the maximum frequency observed in 1000 gene populations. The higher the value obtained, the more likely it is to be harmful. Range of -2 to 3 in dbNSFP.
MetaLR	Prediction mechanism based on logistic regression, which incorporates ten other predictors (SIFT, PolyPhen-2 HDIV, PolyPhen-2 HVAR, GERP++, MutationTaster, Mutation Assessor, FATHMM, LRT, SiPhy, PhyloP) as well as the maximum frequency observed in 1000 gene populations. The higher the result, the more likely it is to be harmful. Range from 0 to 1.
Mutation Advisor	Server capable of predicting the impact of amino acid substitutions in proteins, such as mutations discovered in cancer or *missense* polymorphisms. The functional impact is accessed based on the evolutionary conservation of the affected amino acid in homologous proteins.

In view of these predictors, it is possible to determine with confidence which of the mutations available in the database are drivers and which are passengers. And therefore effectively compare the real data screened with the simulated data acquired.

4.4Statistical analysis - Regression model

We used the coefficient of determination, known as R^2 , because it is information that determines whether the model can explain the observed values. It's a measure based on linear regression and can therefore determine whether the values of our x, number of drivers, are a conditional parameter for estimating the value of our *y,* number of *passengers.* The higher the R^2 the more explanatory the model, the more it fits the sample. Its value is governed by Equation 4 below.

Equation 4 - *R-value*[2] .

$$R^2 = 1 - \frac{SQ_{res}}{SQ_{tot}}$$

In this equation we have that $5Q_{tot}$ is the total sum of squares, i.e. the sum of the squares of the differences between the mean and each observed value, SQ_{res} is the sum of squares of the residuals, which calculates the unexplained part of the model, i.e. values that are not explained by the model. The value of R^2 varies between 0 and 1 and indicates in percentage how well the model can explain the observed values.

CHAPTER 5

RESULTS AND DISCUSSION

This section includes the results obtained in the study. In addition, some points for discussion, which correlate with the results, will also be presented.

5.1 Stochastic Modelling and Simulations

Given the importance of mutations in tumour development, one of the objectives was to analyse whether the time between mutations decreases as the number of mutations increases. We used the branching model because it better represents the biological process of acquiring mutations, making numerical simulations feasible. In the model, at each step, two days, all the cells will either (i) divide without acquiring a new **driver** mutation, (ii) divide acquiring a new **driver** mutation, or (iii) die. The possibility of the cell entering quiescence or differentiating is modelled within the 'death' group. We also assume that *driver* mutations reduce the possibility of cell death.

The parameters listed in Table 3 were used, along with a folding time suitable for breast cancer (2 days). A total of 100,000 simulations were carried out.

Of these, those that only obtained the first *driver* mutation were disregarded (98,951 simulations), i.e. 98.95% of all simulations. Many of these simulations didn't make it to the second step of the simulation and died soon afterwards. This is due to the fact that the probability of cell death is initially higher, since the adaptive advantage of the mutated cell is not high. In turn, it won't be able to survive in the organism unless it achieves a relevant adaptive advantage for its survival. Furthermore, as Bozic himself states, not all simulated mutations are successful because stochastic fluctuations can lead to the extinction of a lineage.

Figure 6 shows the number of simulations obtained per number of *driver* mutations (lineages) in total.

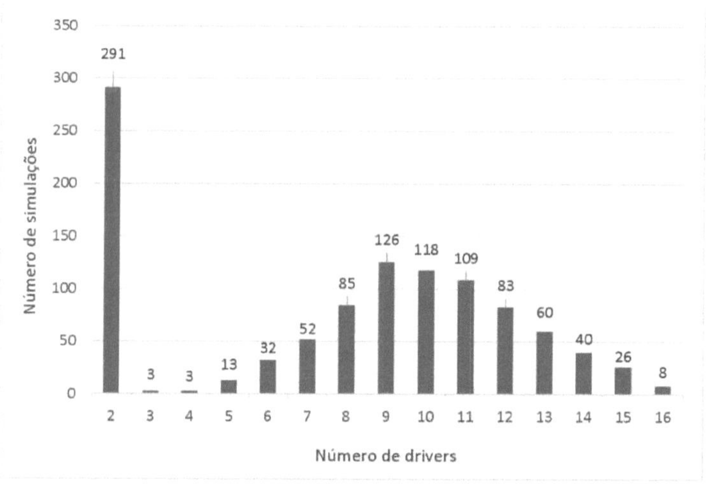

Figure 6 - Number of simulations obtained with the maximum number of *drivers*.

It's interesting to note the distribution of the number of these simulations. Those that obtained only two driver mutations were much more frequent than all the others; but the simulations with three and four drivers were well below expectations. This can be explained by the value of the s parameter, which represents the adaptive advantage. It is likely that once the tumour has acquired a certain number (three or four) of driver mutations, it has already obtained enough adaptive advantage to remain in the organism for longer, thus guaranteeing its survival. We therefore found very few simulations that ended with three or four mutations, as this number of mutations was not yet enough to counterbalance the chance of the lineages going extinct.

Another important point is the also high number of driver mutations, between six and fourteen mutations. Again, this is explained by the high adaptive factor that the cancer cells have already obtained. Once they have acquired enough driver mutations, it is possible to find an increase in the rate of cell cloning, thus accelerating their expansion and making it impossible for the organism to prevent growth through its own mechanisms.

We have chosen some representative images, shown in Figure 7, of population growth based on the number of mutations. In this figure we present eight examples of the simulations, where each colour represents a driver mutation lineage and its population growth behaviour over time. In 7a,

For example, we have a lineage that started and grew rapidly (curve in black), but which after a certain number of iterations was unable to persist and died out shortly after the death of the lineage of two **driver** mutations (dots in red). In the following images we see that after acquiring the limiting number of mutations, around three or four mutations, the tumour grew rapidly over time.

An important observation was found in the simulations shown in figures 7d, 7e, 7f, 7g, 7h, where after a certain amount of simulation time the following lineages exceeded the number of cells in the first lineage. In figure 7b, the second mutation only occurred about 10 years after the initial one, but it only took three years for the third mutation to occur. Figure 8h shows that the new mutations are even annualised after 15 years of simulation. This confirms what was said in Figure 2, which states that with each new mutation the time until the next one decreases and consequently the rate of cell division increases, thus overlapping the number of cells of the following lineages in relation to the initial one.

For the simulation with a total of 16 **driver** mutations (Figure 8h), the total number of cells in the tumour was 6.85 x 10^{17} cells, a figure that has no biological support, since the total number of cells in the body is around $1O^{1Z}$ and 10^{16} (BIANCONI, 2013). This behaviour in the simulation is due to the time and action of the mutations, and could correspond to a highly aggressive tumour, but in practice the aggressiveness of the tumour's action would have already caused the patient's death.

The results presented were based on growth parameters found in the literature, specifically the acquisition rates of **driver** mutations and the folding time specific to breast cancer. Without this, there would be no biological support for comparing the efficacy of the model to that used by Bozic with gliobastoma and pancreatic cancer (BOZIC et al., 2010). By using this approach based on biologically relevant premises, we can evolve from an applied maths model to a mathematical model with prospects for biological applications.

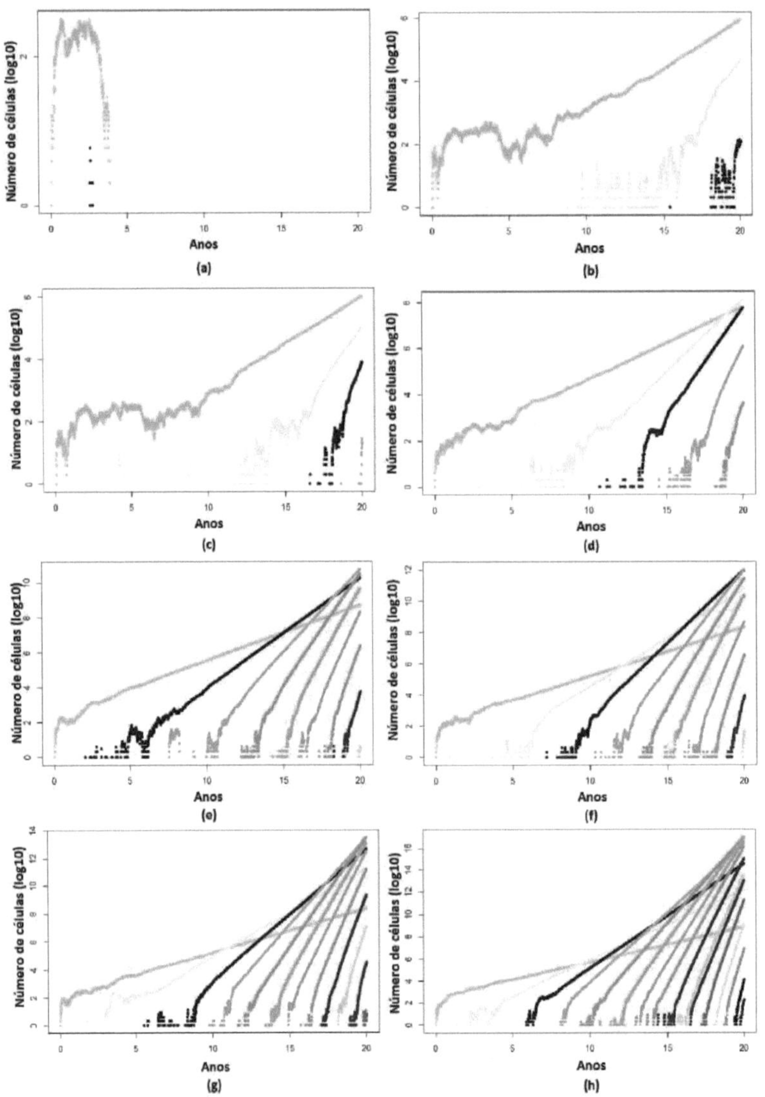

Figure 7 - Representation of the simulations - number of cells per simulation time (tumour age). Each graph represents a realisation of the same stochastic model, using the same parameters and each colour represents a lineage with "n" *driver* mutations. 7a, two *drivers*; 7b, three *drivers*; 7c, four *drivers*; 7d, five *drivers*; 7e, nine *drivers*; 7f, ten *drivers*; 7g, twelve *drivers*; 7h, sixteen *drivers*.

Equation 2 was used to determine the number of **passengers** in the simulations, where **t** is calculated as the number of steps (iterations) from the start of the simulation to the start of the last lineage. The graph in Figure 8 shows a dependence of the growth in the number of **passengers** on the number of **drivers**, and after four **driver** mutations, the number of **passengers** stabilised at 28 to 29 mutations.

It is likely that the method used does not come close enough to biological behaviour, but it can be seen that there is an initial increase in the number of **passenger** mutations in relation to the **drivers**, and that after a certain time the number of mutations stagnates. This suggests that there is a real relationship between the number of **passengers** and their dependence on **driver** mutations. The explanation lies in the fact that **passenger** mutations are nothing more than the product of defective cell multiplication and therefore play no role in the dynamics of tumour growth (neutral mutations). And this accumulation probably occurs because the driver mutations affect some metabolic pathways (acquired capacities of the cancer) that lead to greater cell proliferation, either by increasing the frequency of the cell cycle or by decreasing the cycle time.

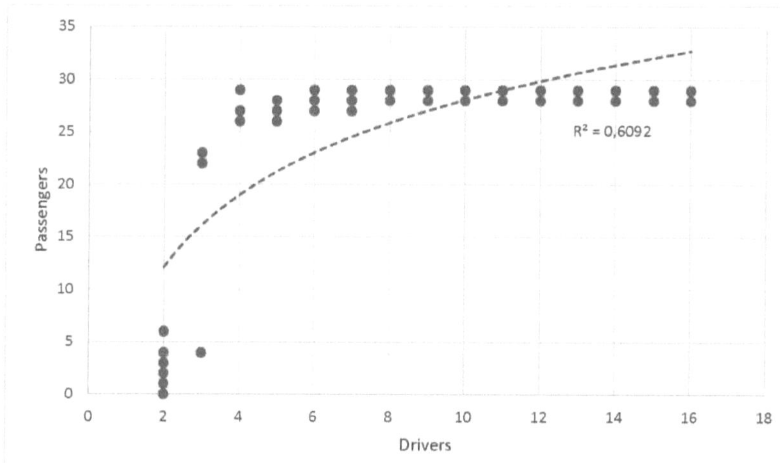

Figure 8 - Number of *passengers* obtained in simulations with maximum number of *drivers*.

Comparing our results with those obtained by Bozic et al. an important point to comment on is that, among the premises considered is that there wasn't much cell division before the tumour started, so we can consider the beginning of everything from the first **driver** mutation. More complete information about breast cancer is difficult to find, such as whether or not there were accumulations of **passenger** mutations before the first **driver** was acquired. In addition, the folding time for breast epithelial cells varies greatly, according to the literature, between 24 and 120h (DAI, 2015), which for the study carried out greatly influences the results.

However, as Bozic states, it is expected that the average adaptive advantage of a **driver** mutation will be similar from the point of view of all tumour types, since the pathways by which these mutations act overlap to a considerable degree. This line of reasoning may be correct looking at Figure 8 where the logarithmic behaviour is maintained for the case of breast cancer. Where the accumulated time to acquire **k** mutations increases logarithmically with **k**.

5.2 Bioinformatics and Genomic Data Analysis

To assess the relevance of the model, we compared the simulation results with information obtained from bioinformatic analysis (DB Mutation data) in relation to the proportion of *passenger* **and** *driver* **mutations. Figures 9 and 10 show the proportions of** *drivers* **and** *passengers* **for breast cancer found in DB Mutation, following the criteria presented in the methodology. Due to certain discrepancies in the data from each bank, around 80% of the samples from TCGA did not pass DB Mutation's classification filters, which is why the data obtained from each bank was analysed separately. In addition, we disregarded samples with many mutations (samples with more than 30 mutations) in order to be more lenient when comparing the data generated from the simulations.**

As we can see, the **passenger/driver** distributions show a similar behaviour to the **passenger/driver** ratio graph from the simulations, where we have a number of samples with few **driver** mutations and, after an interval of few mutations, we again have a concentration of samples in higher numbers for **driver** mutations.

Based on the coefficient of determination R^2 *of the* curve, it can be seen that the data from the COSMIC database is more relevant than that from the TCGA database. The R^2 varies between 0 and 1 and indicates, in percentage, how well the model can explain the observed values. This goes back to the problem we encountered when selecting the samples, where there were discrepancies between the databases, with the aggravating factor that most of the TCGA data was not filtered by the DB Mutation classifiers. Therefore, the data analysed may not provide complete information, since DB Mutation was unable to efficiently classify the information available in the samples. Overcoming this deficiency in both DB Mutation and TCGA will help us in the future to compare simulated data with real data.

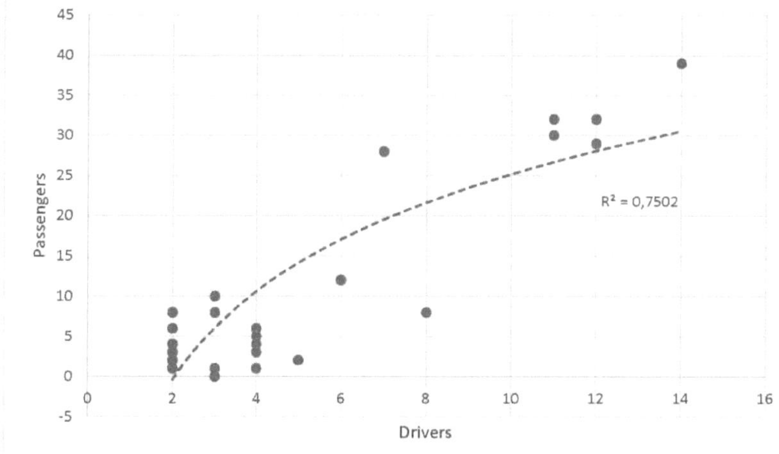

Figure 9 - Proportion of *drivers and passengers* for the COSMIC database.

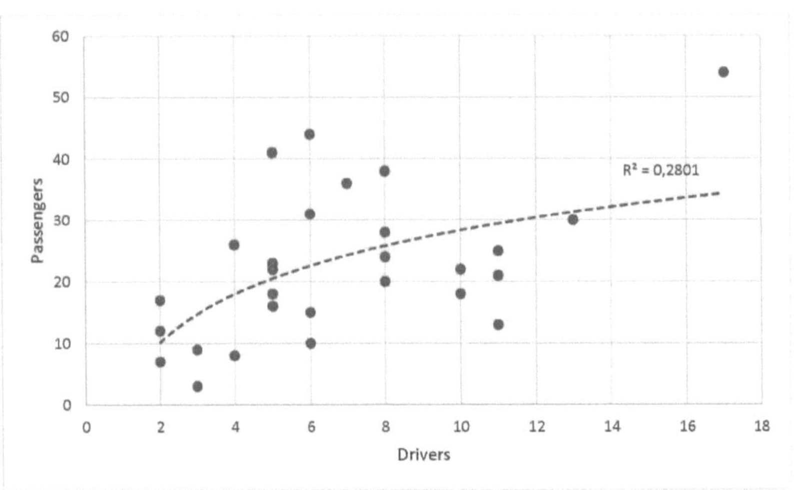

Figure 10 - Proportion of *drivers and passengers* for the TCGA database.

Another comparison to be made with the work carried out by Bozic and colleagues is in the flowchart she used to classify mutations and compare the real data (glioblastoma multiforme and pancreas) with the simulated data. The authors used a simplistic definition to classify mutations in a sample as **drivers**, considering that if the mutation was **missense** it would invariably be a **driver** mutation. This consideration may not be very applicable from a biological point of view, and a more formal definition is needed that does not leave room for false negatives and positives.

However, the predictions she made and her results are also in line with the results obtained during this study. As with all existing models, it is necessary to make limiting assumptions, such as those used in this model, but these assumptions do not fail to provide the key conclusions of the study, which can aid a better understanding of biological processes.

This shows that the real context of the model and its results support enough information to believe that tumours and their growth are dependent on **driver** mutations. In addition, the ratio of **driver** mutations to **passenger** mutations is also dependent and shows logarithmic behaviour.

CHAPTER 6

CONCLUSION

In view of the above, we can understand that the study has achieved its objective of presenting an evolutionary dynamics model and comparatively analysing the simulation results with breast cancer data.

Our results showed that after acquiring driver mutations, the tumour accelerates its process of acquiring new mutations. The time taken to acquire the second mutation was ten years and for the third to cost two. Furthermore, the acquisition of passenger mutations is dependent on tumour growth and consequently on the number of driver mutations it has.

We also observed the logarithmic relationship between the types of mutations, driver and passenger, where after a certain simulation time the number of passenger mutations enters a plateau state, due to the maximum number of possible steps for the defined simulation time. In addition, we proved that the adaptive advantage factor, s, really is a safe parameter for future simulations.

We believe that for the future of research into the evolutionary dynamics of tumours, we must establish parameters that are ever closer to biology, since there are many factors that limit the dynamics.

In the future we will be able to test cancer treatments using simulations and then test them in vivo. However, we understand that there is still a long way to go in terms of modelling the dynamics of tumour growth and the factors that contribute to its development.

CHAPTER 7

REFERENCES

1. **ARMITAGE, Peter; DOLL, Richard. The age distribution of cancer and a multi- stage theory of carcinogenesis. British journal of cancer, v. 8, n. 1, p. 1, 1954.**
2. **BALMAIN, Allan et al. How many mutations are required for tumourigenesis? Implications from human cancer data. Molecular carcinogenesis, v. 7, n. 3, p. 139-146,1993.**
3. **BIOME - MULTIDISCIPLINARY BIOINFORMATICS CENTRE. DB Mutation, 2016. Available at :http://www.bioinformatics-brazil.org/dbmutation/. Accessed on: 26 November 2016.**
4. **BISHOP, J. Michael; WEINBERG, Robert Aliem (Ed.). Scientific American molecular oncology. Scientific American, 1996.**
5. **BOZIC, Ivana et al. Accumulation of driver and passenger mutations during tumour progression. Proceedings of the National Academy of Sciences, v. 107, n. 43, p. 18545-18550, 2010.**
6. **BOZIC, Ivana; ALLEN, Benjamin; NOWAK, Martin A. Dynamics of targeted cancer therapy. Trends in molecular medicine, v. 18, n. 6, p. 311-316, 2012.**
7. **CÁRTER, Hannah et al. Cancer-specific high-throughput annotation of somatic mutations: computational prediction of driver missense mutations. Cancer research, v. 69, n. 16, p. 6660-6667, 2009.**
8. **DAI, Xiaofeng et al. Breast cancer intrinsic subtype classification, clinical use and future trends. American journal of cancer research, v. 5, n. 10, p. 2929, 2015.**

9. DURRETT, Rick et al. Evolutionary dynamics of tumour progression with random fitness values. Theoretical population biology, v. 78, n. 1, p. 54-66, 2010.

10. DURRETT, Rick et al. Intratumour heterogeneity in evolutionary models of tumour progression. Genetics, v. 188, n. 2, p. 461-477, 2011.

11. FOULDS, L. The experimental study of tumour progression: a review. Cancer research, v. 14, n. 5, p. 327-339, 1954.

12. HAHN, William C. et al. Creation of human tumour cells with defined genetic elements. Nature, v. 400, n. 6743, p. 464-468,1999.

13. HANAHAN, Douglas; FOLKMAN, Judah. Pattems and emerging mechanisms of the angiogenic switch during tumourigenesis. cell, v. 86, n. 3, p. 353-364, 1996.

14. HANAHAN, Douglas; WEINBERG, Robert A. The hallmarks of cancer, cell, v. 100, n. l,p. 57-70, 2000.

15. HANAHAN, Douglas; WEINBERG, Robert A. Hallmarks of cancer: the next generation. cell, v. 144, n. 5, p. 646-674, 2011.

16. INSTITUTO NACIONAL DO CÂNCER JOSÉ ALENCAR GOMES DA SILVA. Estimativa 2016 - Incidência do Câncer no Brasil, 2016. Available at: < http://www.inca.gov.br/estimativa/2016/index.asp?ID=2 />. Accessed on: 20 November 2016.

17. LIU, Xiaoming; JIAN, Xueqiu; BOERWINKLE, Eric. dbNSFP v2. 0: a database of human non-synonymous SNVs and their functional predictions and annotations. Human mutation, v. 34, n. 9, p. E2393-E2402, 2013.

18. NOWAK, Martin A. Evolutionary dynamics. Harvard University Press, 2006.

19. **R CORE TEAM. R: A language and environment for statistical computing. R Foundation for Statistical Computing, Vienna, Austria. Available at: <http://www.R-project.org/>. Accessed on: 26 November 2016.**

20. **REGOES, Roland R. Population genetics meets cancer genomics. Proceedings of the National Academy of Sciences, v. 107, n.43,p. 18241-18242, 2010.**

21. **STEWART, B. et al. World cancer report 2014. World, 2016.**

22. **STRATTON, Michael R.; CAMPBELL, Peter J.; FUTREAL, P. Andrew. The cancer genome. Nature, v. 458, n. 7239, p. 719-724, 2009.**

23. **THE SCIENTIST. Combing the Cancer Genome, 2012. Available at: http://www.the-scientist.com/7articles.view/articleNo/31747/title/Combing-the- Cancer-Genome/. Accessed on: 05 December 2016.**

24. **WACLAW, Bartlomiej et al. A spatial model predicts that dispersai and cell tumover limit intratumour heterogeneity. Nature, v. 525, n. 7568, p. 261-264, 2015.**

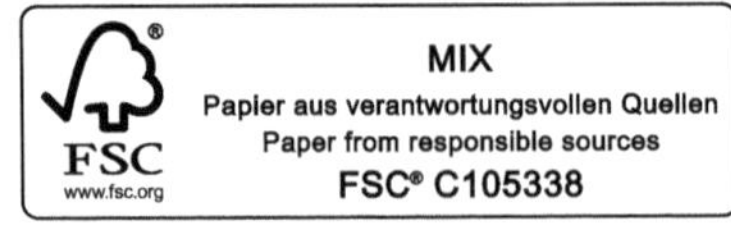

Printed by Books on Demand GmbH, Norderstedt / Germany